HOW TO TALK DIRTY

354 Hottest Dirty Talk Examples to Bring Your

Wildest Fantasies and Deepest Desires to Life

DISCLAIMER

This disclaimer applies to any damages or injury caused by the use and application, whether directly or indirectly, of any advice or information presented, whether for breach of contract, tort, negligence, personal injury, criminal intent, or under any other cause of action. You are responsible for your own choices, actions, and results.

LEGAL NOTICE

Upon using the information contained in this book, you agree to accept all risks of using the information presented inside this book and to hold harmless the Author from and against any damages, costs, and expenses, including any legal fees potentially resulting from the application of any of the information provided by this guide. No liability is assumed for losses or damages due to the information provided.

WARNING

The content and vocabulary in this book is intended for ages 18+. It may contain adult subject matter including explicit sexual content.

CONTENTS

INTRODUCTION

Sex is great, but if you're like many people, it's even better with a little dirty talk. Whether you like to give or get, dirty talk can be exciting and it turns an ordinary sexual encounter into something really amazing.

You've probably picked up this book for one of two reasons: you enjoy dirty talk, but aren't sure how to get started or feel embarrassed about it, or you want to expand your repertoire of bawdy phrases and spice things up a bit more.

How to Use This Book

These pages are full of dirty talk, from simple phrases that let your lover know that you want them, to far more descriptive options that let them know exactly what you intend to do with them. It's up to you to choose what level of naughty you want to use, but if you're new to this, it's a good idea to start out with the milder phrases.

Flip to the section that best suits your needs (male, female, unisex, etc.) and pick a level of dirty that fits what you're comfortable with. Then start reading. You can choose a couple of phrases to use the next time you're getting hot and heavy with someone special, just to try them out.

Don't just memorize everything in this book. While there are plenty of great examples of words and sentences you can use, these aren't meant to be repeated just as you read them. Add your own twist and make them your own. If you like to use the word "shaft" instead of "dick," go ahead and substitute it. Switch up body parts and focus on what YOU like.

In short, this is the book to inspire you and get you going with talking dirty, but it shouldn't be the only resource you use. Your mind is even more powerful and once you've read through the appropriate sections here, you'll have a much better library of erotic phrasings in your head that can be used whenever you like.

EXPANDING YOUR NAUGHTY VOCABULARY

One of the biggest problems with dirty talk is sounding repetitious. If you find that you're just repeating the same word over and over, you might need to look into expanding your vocabulary. While there are complete phrases further on in the book, you can mix them up a bit by substituting different words as you desire.

For example, if the phrase is "I want your dick inside me." You can easily switch it out to say, "I want your prick/rod/cock inside me."

Aroused: chubbed, horny, hot and bothered, hot and ready, soaked, turned on, wet

Anus: arsehole, asshole, backdoor, back end, bang hole, brown eye, brown star, bunghole, butt hole, chocolate starfish, cornhole, Hershey Highway, o-ring, poop chute, puckered brown eye

Breasts: boobs, boobies, bust, chest puppies, fun bags, gazongas, girls, hooters, jugs, melons, mosquito bites, naughty pillows, rack, tatas, tits, titties, the twins

Clitoris: Bean, button, clit, devil's doorbell, fun button, happy button, hooded lady, kernel, love bud, love button, man in the boat, nub, sweet spot

Ejaculate: blast, blow your load, blow your wad, bust, bust a nut, bust a wad, climax, cream, cum, get your nut off, jizz, nut, pop, shoot, shoot your load, splooge, spurt, squirt

Erection: boner, chubby, get it up, hard-on, stiffy, tent pole, wood

Have sex: bang, be intimate, boink, bone, breed, doing it, doing the nasty, frig, fuck, get busy, get down, get it on, get laid, get some, go balls-deep, hanky panky, hot beef injection, hump, jump bones, knock boots, lay pipe, make love, make whoopee, mate, mish, nail, pork, pound, roll in the hay, rut, score, screw, sex, tap ass

Masturbate: beat it, beat off, beat your meat, choke the chicken, crack one off, fab, flick your bean (women), flog your log, have a wank, jack off, jerk off, jerk the gherkin, jill (women), jill off (women), play with yourself, polish your knob, rub one off, slap the salami, spank it, spank the monkey, stroke it, toss, toss off, tug, wack off, wank, wank off

Oral Sex (Male): beej, BJ, blow, blow job, bob on a knob, buff, deep throat, give/get head, head, hoover, hummer, nosh, slurp the gherkin, suck, suck dick, suck off, swallow

Oral Sex (Female): eat a peach, eat out, give face, go down on, go downtown, have a box lunch, muff dive, munch carpet, nosh, oral, lick

Penis: baby maker, cock, dick, love stick, love shaft, one eyed monster, pecker, pole, prick,, rod, schlong, shaft, trouser snake, wang, willy

Semen: baby batter, baby gravy, cream, cum, ghost load, jizm, jizz, load, man chowder, man seed, nut, pole milk, seed, splooge, wad

Testicles: balls, ball sack, bollocks, boys, coin purse, cojones, family jewels, grapes, nads, nuggets, nuts, nut sack

Vagina: bang hole, beaver, cooch, cunny, cunt, flower, fuck hole, love cave, love taco, muff, muffin, pookie, poontang, pooter, pussy, quif, quim, slit, snatch, vag

Some of these words may feel silly or ridiculous to you, and that's fine! Pick what works for you and what you're comfortable with, then start using them.

GETTING STARTED WITH DIRTY TALK

Dirty talk might seem like something . . . well, dirty, so it can take a bit to get started. If you know you want to be one of those people who can sling out naughty words whenever you're feeling a little horny, this book will help. But first, you need to garner the confidence to start.

Does your mind go blank when you're in the act? Then here's something to consider . . . try just describing what you're doing or what is being done to you.

For example, you might say, "I love fucking you." Or maybe "It feels amazing when you suck on my cock like that." Describe what is going on and what you like about it. This is a nice easy way to start out.

Not everyone is comfortable with naughtier terms and that's fine. Start with what comes naturally to you and then work in a few new words every so often. Eventually, they'll become second nature and you'll be dirty talking like a pro.

Seduction: The Art of Dirty Talk in Foreplay

Did you know that talking dirty can start long before you actually have sex? Texting and talking on the phone, or even just sending your special someone off with a naughty phrase in the morning can get your engines revving!

Anticipation is the best foreplay there is. When you let your lover know that there is something special awaiting them when they get home tonight, they'll be thinking about it all day long. You just need to let them know what you're thinking early enough in the day that it will get them hot and bothered long before they're home.

A good way to start with this, is just to tell your partner how sexy they look before they head out for the day. You can also text them to let them know you're thinking of them, or even to send a list of things you plan to do to them later. Just be sure to send this sort of thing in a private message, not a work email or something that others could see!

Describe what you want to do to their body, tell them how horny you are and how you just can't wait to fuck them. Or go a little more subtle and tell your partner that you're touching yourself thinking about them and you're not sure you can hold off until you see each other again.

Foreplay doesn't have to just involve touching. It can also be very mental and dirty talk is the perfect way to make it happen.

Getting Down and Dirty

Once you're in bed, it may become easier to talk dirty. You'll find that the more aroused you both are, the easier the words tumble from your lips. The following tips will help you speak up like a pro.

Be Confident

Timidly murmuring that you want to fuck someone into oblivion doesn't really work, so go into this with all the confidence you can muster. You know you're sexy and your partner is, too, so now is the perfect time to let that shine.

It's usually best to start out with some mild compliments and work up to the nastier stuff, particularly if you are with a new person. You don't know how they might react and it could end up being a bit much for them. This is particularly true when it comes to men dirty talking to women. It can come across as a bit creepy if you jump straight into calling her a bitch and a whore or slut.

Watch Your Lover

Is your partner into dirty talk? Most people are, to a certain extent, but you need to observe to see what exactly turns them on. They might start talking dirty right back, which is a great indication that they love it. However, you might not hear any words, but body language says a lot, too. Signs your lover is getting off on your dirty talk include:

- Faster breathing
- Moaning
- Arching the back
- Touching themselves
- Gasps

- Faster sexual rhythm

Body language says a lot, so once you know what your lover likes, you can do a lot more of it. If they're not responding favorably, you may need to switch to something a little less aggressive.

Fantasize with Them

This is the perfect time to share your fantasies and get creative about what you want to do to your lover. You may even find that you are both into the same fantasies, so go ahead and talk it out, making your ideas into something sexy and invigorating.

You may even want to take the next step and actually act out your fantasies, but that's a topic for another book. For now, just talk about it and discuss what you would do to your lover in different hypothetical situations. For example, if you were in a crowded nightclub and no one noticed that you were getting it on, how would you touch the other person?

Start Slow and Build

Good dirty talk doesn't leap straight into the nastiest talk right away. Start out slowly with things like, "I want you so bad right now." Then build up to the harder options. You should know exactly what kind of things your partner wants to hear, too. You may not be able to build up to the filthy phrases listed further on in this book, because your partner just isn't into it.

That being said, as you get hornier and more into what you're doing, you'll find it easier and easier to talk dirty, because your brain is focused more on what you're doing. Arousal can do amazing things to the human brain. Your partner is more likely to be turned on by things they wouldn't consider when not aroused, too.

Use the Force

The hornier you both are, the easier it will be to talk dirty and to listen to dirty talk. If you think about it, you've probably tried a few things in the heat of the moment that you would never do when you weren't insanely turned on.

The same goes for dirty talk. So, once you are getting busy and are totally turned on, it's the perfect time to start smack talking and showing your lover just what you're made of.

There's also less chance of rejection or laughter in the middle of sex, because you're both feeling it and the sexual force is strong. In fact, you might get some dirty talk right back.

Practice Makes Perfect

Like all things worth doing, dirty talk requires plenty of practice and you need to keep trying. Talk dirty to your partner whenever you have a chance. Do it during sex, over the phone, and in texts. The more you do, the better you'll get!

If you're really shy, you can always practice on your own. This works best if you're getting off as you talk, but you can also practice in front of a mirror. Either way, the phrases should start to fall off your tongue.

Choose Your Pet Names

It can feel really awkward to suddenly start saying, "Oh god, baby, yes," when you've never called your lover baby before. For some people, coming up with the right pet names can be the most important part of preparing for dirty talk.

You might want to stick to the basics, like baby, honey, lover, etc. or you can take things a step further and call your lover daddy, love slave, master, mistress, etc. If you really want to get nasty, bitch, whore, cum slut, bastard, and similar labels can be used. Keep in mind that not everyone enjoys being called a slut, so gauge your audience before going too far with this one.

Sex is amazing and can be a lot of fun, but dirty talk really elevates it to the next level. Not everyone will try talking dirty, but they're really missing out on something incredible. Go ahead and try it out for yourself and find out what you're comfortable with and what your lover likes, too. You might be surprised.

UNISEX PHRASES

The dirty talk in this section applies to either gender and can be a fun way to spice up your sex life. If you're just getting started, aim for the milder phrases, but feel free to add in your own wording or move on to the hotter phrases as you feel ready.

You can use these different ideas for sexy talk to create your own hot lines, as well. The trick here is to get creative. Just use what is listed below as inspiration.

Mild Dirty Talk

These phrases are easy to start out with and will help get you in the mood for a little hanky panky. Used well, they can help you feel even sexier and turn on your partner, too.

I want you.

You can spice this one up later by adding where you want them, what you want them to do, or even just adding a couple of curse words. For example, "I fucking want you between my legs."

You're so hot/sexy.

Nothing like a good, sexy compliment to turn someone on!

I love every inch of your body.

Let your lover know just how much you enjoy their body by starting out with this phrase and then launching into what you like about each part.

We fit so perfectly together.

This is ideally said as you come together the first time, but can work at any point during sex.

You need to take those clothes off right now.

Want your lover naked? Tell them to strip. You can either help or watch and make it a sexy strip show.

You turn me on/make me horny.

Again, everyone likes to hear that they have a sexual effect on their partner, so this can be a good one to break out early on.

The way you smell/look/taste/feel drives me wild.

Pick a sense and run with it . . . or use multiples in the same compliment.

You can stay, but the clothes gotta go.

This is a simple ultimatum that will result in sexier times quickly.

We really should be filming this.

When you're this good together, it really should be captured on film for the world (or just you two) to see.

You are the best lay I've ever had.

Put your lover up on a pedestal and make sure they know just how amazing they actually are.

Making you horny is one of my favorite things to do.

Let there be no doubt that you live to please. This is a fun way to start the dirty talk off with your loved one.

I love how you smell/taste/feel.

Similar to the previous phrase, this lets you expound on what your senses are noting about your lover's body.

You make me feel so good.

This phrase can be used during foreplay, or sex, or even after the act, since it lets the person know just how you feel about what they're doing.

Tease me until I'm begging for it.

If you enjoy being teased, this is the perfect way to go about getting your partner to do it.

You better be naked when I get home.

On your way back home? Make sure you let your partner know what to expect when you get back. This is a great text message to send.

God, I love how you feel against me.

These words are perfect for dirty talking after sex, or during . . . so get creative.

Our bodies were made for each other. They fit perfectly.

This can be used during sex or even just with a cuddle, where her head tucks perfectly under your chin. It's romantic and sexy.

I'm going to make you feel so good.

You can use this phrase any time, referring to future sex acts, but it's particularly powerful when you text it or say it when you are planning to meet up soon.

The way you walk/cook/talk turns me on so much.

Whatever your partner is doing, let them know that they turn you on by doing it. This is a good way to turn an ordinary task into sexy time.

I just want to do this forever.

Enjoying whatever you're doing to your lover? Let them know how incredible it is by sharing your desire to keep going forever.

I could lie here/cuddle you forever like this.

Give that special someone a good indication that you're enjoying yourself, even if you haven't made it to the actual act yet. This phrase also works as pillow talk, after the fact.

You have no idea how much you/your body turn(s) me on.

Just telling them this will usually give your partner an idea of how sexy you find them, but it will also turn them on.

You're amazing.

Who doesn't want to hear that they're incredible? Both male and female partners will love hearing this.

You taste like _____.

Add in something wonderful, like honey, vanilla, etc. to make your lover swoon. This is also helpful if they are feeling a little shy about oral sex.

You drive me crazy when you _____.

Pick something that your lover does that you enjoy and encourage them to do it more often by using this phrase to let them know.

Your _____ is/are so beautiful.

Choose a body part you like and let your partner know just what you think of it. They'll be thrilled and it will turn them on more. Not sure which body part to focus on? Eyes, lips, and necks are always a good start.

Shut up and just kiss me.

Giving a command can be a turn on for both parties, so get creative and tell your partner what you want them to do.

I'm making the rules/in control tonight.

While this might not sound dirty, it can be very exciting to take control. This phrase also lets you take things a step further with commands after it.

Cancel everything you planned tonight. Tonight you're mine.

Take charge and make some serious plans to steam the place up with this kind of dirty talk.

As you wish.

Who wouldn't love to have a genie grant their every wish? While you may not be a genie, you can certainly make your partner feel amazing by following their commands.

You make me feel so good.

Your lover will strive to make you feel even better when they hear this.

Oh baby, you're the best.

This is a nice simple phrase that will definitely get them roused. Better yet, they'll try to improve on their past record.

Come make love to me. I need you.

Make love is a pretty gentle way to talk about sex and can feel more familiar if you're new to dirty talk.

How did I get so lucky?

Take this one up a step by describing what is so incredible about your lover, from their eyes, to their sexy bits.

Oh, god, that feels so good!

Sometimes, keeping it simple is all that's needed. Just let your lover know what feels good and they'll do more of it.

You're going to make me cum already.

Nothing says "you're sexy" like telling your partner that they're going to make you come fast.

That's perfect, keep it up.

Like what they're doing? Then tell them so they'll keep going!

Tell me you're mine.

If you find that you enjoy hearing dirty talk, but your partner is shy, you can tell them what to say.

I want to explore every nook and cranny of your body.

Say this and then start doing it for maximum effect. Use lips, fingers, etc. to do the exploring and keep it sexy.

I can't handle not being able to touch you.

If you're not able to be together part of the time, this phrase will make the other person hotter for you than ever.

I never knew I could want someone this much.

If your partner is making you feel things you never felt before, go ahead and tell them so they can enjoy feeling special.

Your lips are irresistible.

While you can start by complimenting their lips, don't forget that other body parts can also be irresistible and don't be afraid to expand on that.

Do you even realize what you do to me?

If they don't know what they do to you, it's time to tell them
. . . going into great detail.

I'll do whatever you want, just tell me when and where.

Having you completely to themselves, with the ability to tell
you exactly what to do to their body is something that most
lovers will cherish. And take full advantage of.

Dirty Talk

Are you beyond the basics? Then you'll want to get a little sexier and a little dirtier. The phrases given here are a good stepping stone to being really sexy. They are a bit harsher for those who are sensitive to sex talk, though, so you want to be sure that your partner is okay with this kind of dirty talk.

Where do you want me to make you cum?

Turn the reins over to the other person, while letting them know exactly what you have in mind for them.

You look good in that outfit. Now take it off.

Clothes don't really matter when you want to make love to someone, so get them naked faster with dirty talk.

I haven't been this horny since I first discovered masturbating.

If your lover makes you feel like a teenager again, then you definitely need to share this bit of information to make them feel as sexy as you see them.

Bite me right there.

Get a bit raunchy with some biting and roughness added into your foreplay. All you need to do is tell them what to do.

I love making/watching you cum.

Your lover might be a bit shy about cumming, but this is a great way to reassure them that you enjoy watching.

Cumming together is the best part.

Plan to cum as a couple by riling your partner up as you get closer to orgasm. While it doesn't always work, the orgasm will still be incredible.

I need a good fuck right now, you up for it?

Whether it's stress or you're just horny as heck, get them on your side and have some great sex together.

I want to cum for you so hard.

Of course, this is only possible if your partner makes you cum, so this is a good reminder that they need to get busy.

You're the hottest fuck ever.

Without directly comparing, let your lover know that you have never been with anyone this hot and sexy.

You feel so sexy to me.

Right now, in this moment, this person is the sexiest being alive. It's the perfect time to go ahead and make them aware of it.

How bad do you want to cum for me?

Take control and make them beg for it . . . by telling you how much they want to cum.

I've been naughty, you better give me a spanking.

An oldie, but a goodie . . . spankings are always in style and you probably do need to be punished.

Everything you do with your tongue is incredible.

This is a great way to make them do more with their tongue, so go ahead and let them know what you're enjoying.

You've been bad and now you're going to get a spanking.

This simply reverses the previous phrase and turns you into the protagonist and assigned punisher.

I've never gotten so turned on just by kissing someone.

Feeling the heat as you kiss that special someone? Let them know with this handy phrase.

You can have me any way you want right now.

Open up the floor to new ideas with this phrase. It lets your partner come up with some of their more interesting methods of having sex and presenting them.

Oh yes, keep doing that!

If you like what your lover is doing, be sure to tell them so they know not to stop.

No one has ever turned me on like you do.

Be sure to let your partner know that you find them super sexy by complimenting them on their ability to turn you on.

Don't stop!

Sometimes the simplest phrase is the best and this one is short and to the point. It's something you can gasp out just before you cum, without expending too much energy.

You can relax, I'm going to do all the work this time/tonight.

After a long day, your lover deserves to be pleasured and it can be fun to tease them by not allowing any "work" on their part at all.

I can still smell you on me and it's wonderful.

Love that sexy scent of your lover? Let them know. This works very well as a text later in the day after you've spent a night together.

I'm coming.

Let the other person know that you're reaching orgasm and it can stimulate them to finish at the same time.

I'm so horny, get over here and make me cum.

Describing how you feel and what you want is a surefire way to make your partner horny, too!

I can't wait to taste you.

These words really get the blood flowing, for both partners, imagining what is to come.

I want your hands on me right now.

When you just can't wait, it helps to communicate that. Your partner will be turned on faster, too.

Eye contact with you is all the foreplay I need.

If you get turned on just looking at your lover, then this is the line for you.

Cum for me, baby.

Just telling someone to cum can be the catalyst for a shocking orgasm. Worth a try, right?

You are a sex fantasy come to life.

Anyone would love to hear this being said about them and it's a good way to butter them up for getting into bed with you.

I want your lips on every part of my body.

This is a perfectly unisex phrase that will have your lover licking and kissing you from top to bottom.

You're so sexy when you cum.

This phrase can be used during orgasm or directly after, particularly if you're still coupled.

Tell me all the dirty things you want to do to me.

Encourage your lover to start talking dirty, too! If they're a bit reluctant, this will give them the motivation to get going.

I'm trying to listen to you, but you're just too damn sexy.

If you can't concentrate on anything but that hot body, then you should probably say so and let them know why you're ignoring them.

I can't stop thinking about your taste on my tongue.

Continue this line of thought with some suggestions on how you can get a taste of those flavors again, preferably sooner rather than later.

I'm going to rip those clothes off you and throw you on the bed.

Not sure what to say? Tell them what you're going to do to them and they'll immediately get hornier.

I'm addicted to your body against mine.

There's no better addiction to have and this one will heat things up considerably.

I want to make you scream in pleasure.

What are you going to do to make them scream? That's the question that will have your lover writhing under you.

Keep this up and I'm going to fucking explode.

This is always a good way to get someone to keep doing what they're doing and maybe even speed it up a bit, in order to make you cum harder.

I always get what I want and I want you.

Take control with this simple, yet very sexy phrase.

You make me want to be very, very bad.

Next, explore just how bad you can get with each other . . . through dirty talk, sexy actions, and anything else you can think of.

Keep the lights on so I can see you while we fuck.

Sometimes it's sexier with the lights on, so get used to doing it in full daylight.

Filthy Phrases

Sometimes, you just need to be more intense than, "I love it when you make love to me." In those cases, you'll want to turn the dial up to 10 with some of the following phrases. Again, this kind of talk is not for everyone, so keep an eye on your partner to gauge their reaction. Sometimes it just takes one thing to really turn them on.

I'm going to fuck you so hard we wake the neighbors.

Urge your lover to make some noise while you go at it with this sexy phrasing.

Let's fuck so hard we break the bed.

This gets expectations up for some seriously hard sex. If you're looking for rough, lead with this.

Let's go to the movies and screw our brains out in the back row.

Remember when you were teenagers and that dark back row was the only place you could get to second base? Take it a step further now that you're older.

I don't care if someone hears, I'm too horny to wait.

If you have a touch of voyeur in you, this particular phrase will be really exciting and it can be for your partner, too.

Get ready, I'm going to fuck your brains out.

This sets the tone for a wild ride and one that is bound to be enjoyable.

Fuck me like you paid for it.

If you want to be treated like a whore or a hustler, then this is the phrase to get your lover really going at it.

Let's do it like we're auditioning for a porn movie.

This gives both of you free reign to be as crazy sexy as you want and it is only bound to turn you both on even more.

Let's fuck until we pass out.

What could be better than fucking each other senseless? Not much, so get on it.

I want to fuck you in front of the mirror.

There's something extra hot about watching yourselves having sex and a mirror is the perfect way to do that.

You are so fucking sexy in that position.

Love this particular position? Make it a favorite by talking dirty about it. You can add exactly what you love about the position (easy access to a body part, etc.).

Tell me how much you want me to fuck you.

This is a great way to get your lover to start talking dirty, too, especially if they're reluctant.

Don't make a sound until I say you can or I'll stop fucking you until you're quiet again.

Commands can be super sexy and trying not to moan is a good way to amp things up a little.

This is going to be the filthiest night of your life.

Whether you're looking at plain old sex or are planning to spice it up a bit, these words will get her wondering what you have in mind.

Don't you dare cum until I say you can.

Again, dominance can be super sexy and once you've said not to come, that's all your partner will be thinking about.

I'm going to make you cum so hard the whole street will know my name.

Planning on a really hard night of fucking? Then this is a good way to start off, by setting expectations.

DIRTY PHRASES FOR MEN

Dirty talk may come more naturally to men, but that doesn't mean they don't need a little inspiration now and then. This section has some handy ideas to get you started with making your woman feel sexy and turned on. You can also use these phrases to let her know that you admire and appreciate her, keeping her mind on the act.

Mild Dirty Talk

The phrases in this part are suitable for any sexual partner and will make her feel amazing. They're mild enough that you don't run the risk of offending your partner, but they still have an effect. She's going to get wet just listening to you talk.

Just looking at you makes me hard.

Let her know she's sexy and beautiful by telling her exactly how it affects your body and she'll want to increase that reaction.

Put an end to my misery . . . open those beautiful legs for me.

She'll feel gorgeous and admired when you say something like this to her.

You're so wet for me.

Sometimes, observations are the best way to go and this is an easy one, if she's as turned on as you are.

I'd turn on some music, but your sexy moans are way better.

Give her permission to get loud by telling her how much you enjoy listening to her express her satisfaction.

Let's skip dessert, I only want you.

Need to get her out of the restaurant fast? Use this phrase to let her know exactly what you are planning.

I've been thinking about your body all day long.

Let her know that you have her on your mind all day and she'll feel extra special.

Wanna bet on how many orgasms I can give you tonight?

Who doesn't love a man who strives for multiple orgasms for his lady? This is the best way to make her wet fast.

Just holding you makes me hard.

She has a major effect on your body and you should tell her all about it.

When you lick your lips like that, I can't handle it.

She'll be licking her lips even more after this and every time, she'll think of how hard it makes you.

I'm going to make you scream in pleasure tonight.

She'll be anticipating an amazing night. This phrase is best said early in the day to get her thinking about it all day long.

You're so tight!

She'll feel amazing when you compliment her on how tight she is and how hard her pussy grips your dick.

When you bend over, I can't control myself.

Let her know how much you appreciate her ass when you tell her that you lose it when she bends over . . . and get ready for a lot more bending.

I can't wait to get you naked on my bed.

This is a good way to let her know just what you have planned for later on in the day. Again, it's helpful to let her know early that you're planning to sex her up at night.

My hands are itching to touch you.

She's going to be itching to be touched after you tell her this. This phrase works well as a text or over the phone.

That sound you made last time we were together is on repeat in my mind.

Do you love her seductive little moans and whimpers when you're together? Then let her know. If she's shy about dirty talk, this is a good way to start moving her toward it.

That sexy ass is begging for a smack.

If you enjoy spanking, this can be a great way to introduce her to the idea. Her reaction will indicate what you should do next.

How is it possible for you to be so sexy and cute at the same time?

Make her feel special when you let her know that you've noticed she's adorable and hot at the same time.

Come here, I'm going to show you who's boss.

This can be a warning or a turn on, really. It's also a great way to start off with some gentle spanking and foreplay.

Fuck, your tits are amazing.

This can be made to sound sexier or less dirty if you like, but the sentiment remains the same.

What a sexy little ass you have.

You can substitute any body part for ass. Just pick what you love best about her and tell her all about it. You can describe her body, too.

Play with your tits for me.

If you enjoy watching her touch herself, you might need to tell her right out what to do. You can also tell her to touch herself downtown, but it's up to you. Most women are more comfortable touching their breasts in front of someone than actively masturbating.

Are you trying to be a cock tease or does it just come naturally?

If she's teasing you and not giving up the goods, this is a good way to find out just what is going on, while sound hot.

I want those legs straight in the air for me.

Sometimes it's best to just tell her straight out what you want from her so you can both enjoy the sex even more.

Get on your stomach/belly.

Direct her to the perfect position for what you have in mind. You can combine this with physically flipping her over.

I want you grinding up against me right now.

It doesn't even have to be sex to be dirty and this phrase will have her rubbing all over you in anticipation of what's to come.

I love feeling your soft skin against me.

Encourage even more touching by complimenting her soft, sexy skin.

Look how hard you make me.

She'll definitely want to look and probably feel you, too. This can be a good intro to sexier talk.

I hope you slept well last night, because you're going to need all your energy tonight.

When you have big plans for pleasing her, it's only fair to let her know ahead of time so she can be prepared.

Your nipples are as hard as my dick.

Pointing out signs of arousal in both of you can only result in the inevitable. You can also try to make her nipples even harder with a little extra work.

Dirty Talk

Ready to take it up a notch? These phrases go beyond teasing and give more explicit pictures in your mind. Use them to turn your partner on and get her riled up and ready for you. These are some phrases that will definitely turn up the heat and may not be for everyone's taste.

You've been dreaming about riding me all day, haven't you?

If she wasn't thinking about it before, she sure is after you say this!

As soon as you walk in, I'm pinning you to the wall and taking what's mine.

What's yours is her pussy, of course, and knowing what's in store for her will make her wetter than she's ever been on her way home.

I want to spank your ass for being too sexy!

This is a great way to start out with a little spanking and make it super hot by talking about what you're doing and why.

Your pussy is like Disneyland for my mouth.

The ultimate compliment, particularly if she's into Disney. But don't just say it, show her exactly what you mean.

I've got whipped cream and chocolate sauce, which one do you want to eat off my dick?

Food play can be particularly sexy and this gives her a choice of what she prefers to lick off your body. Of course, you can flip this around and ask what she wants you to lick off her.

Get your ass in the air and let me slap it.

Position her the way you want and take full advantage of the position. Just telling her what you want will help her get hornier.

I can't wait to slide inside you and hold you in my arms.

If you're separated, for the day or more, you can easily build the anticipation with a little sexy talk via message or phone.

You want me to fill your pussy? Tell me more.

Encourage her to start dirty talking by making her ask for your dick in her pussy. It will turn you both on.

I love watching those titties bounce while you ride my hard dick.

Urge her to move even more and make you feel even better while she's riding you. Bonus, you'll see more bounce than ever.

I'm going to bend you over and make you moan/scream.

Tell her what you're about to do, then go ahead and do it . . . and listen for the moans.

Are you a bad little girl? Do you need to be spanked?

The bad girl theme is an old one, but it's a good one to use, especially if you want an excuse to get a little rough.

Tell me what you've been doing, you naughty girl. I'm going to punish you.

It's up to you to choose the punishment, but this is a good way to lead up to it. Kind of like a really sexy confession.

I love seeing your hands wrapped around my hard cock.

Give her even more reason to touch you by letting her know how incredible it is to see her holding your dick.

I don't think your pussy can handle this dick right now.

Give her a reason to say yes, it can. This is best used while teasing her with your penis rubbing across her without actual penetration. Make her beg for you to come inside.

Touch yourself. I'm just going to watch.

You can learn a lot about what pleasures a woman if you get her to masturbate in front of you, so go ahead and try this line.

Your pussy is mine, all mine.

Claim her body with words and action.

That little quim is in big trouble now.

Has she been naughty? Use this phrase to let her know that she has some serious punishment coming her way.

Let's see who can make who cum first.

This is perfect for 69, with each of you working to make the other orgasm first. It's a win-win situation, really.

I'm going to suck your tits while I fuck the bejeezus out of you.

This phrase will certainly turn her on, since she'll be getting dual sensations and that's always exciting.

This cunny needs to be punished and I have just the dick for the job.

Has she been naughty? Give her a reason for your upcoming punishment.

I want your mouth wrapped around my dick/pole/cock.

This serves as a command and a turn on at the same time. It lets her know exactly what you're looking for and creates an image that is arousing to both of you.

Spread those legs for me.

Get her ready and waiting by giving some simple commands that are bound to turn her on.

Your pussy/cunt tastes amazing.

Let her know that oral sex is just as good for you as it is for her and put her at ease by telling her how great she tastes.

If we weren't in public, I'd be fucking you against this wall/over this table.

Nothing is quite as exciting as alluding to sex in public, even if it's not actually something you would ever do. Just talking about it can be a great bit of foreplay.

We can watch a movie, but you might not be able to concentrate with my mouth on your clit.

The anticipation of an amazing time can really spice things up, so get creative and make sure you share your thoughts with her.

Your juices taste so sweet.

Describe how she tastes (in positive terms, of course) to really make her writhe.

You're going to wake up with my mouth on your pussy.

Give her something to anticipate before you fall asleep and she'll stay wet all night long.

I've had a hard-on all day, just thinking about your hot little body.

She's going to love hearing that you have been thinking of her all this time and it's a surefire way to make her horny, too.

Mmm, I love it when you grind your clit against me.

Give her permission to give herself pleasure, too. After all, nothing is sexier than a woman who knows what she wants.

Don't cum until I say you can. I want to cum with you.

It's hot to orgasm together and it can become a fun way to power play, as well. Of course, as soon as you say not to cum, that's all she can think about!

I want to feel your soft lips on every part of my body.

This very simple phrase gives way to all sorts of imaginings and she'll quickly come up with ways to put her lips to good use.

I want to go down on you all night long.

For any woman who enjoys oral sex, this sentence instantly makes you someone she wants to keep around, so spoil her and watch what happens.

This pussy always gets so wet for me.

Let her know that you've noticed exactly how horny she is for you.

Your lips look so sexy, wrapped around my shaft.

Enjoy the sight of your woman sucking you off? Then let her know by telling her right out how very sexy you find it.

Get on your knees and suck my cock.

Giving commands can be sexy and dominant and will make her swoon. Tell her what you want her to do, but don't forget to let her lay down the rules another day.

Show me how you cum, baby.

Encourage her to masturbate for you by asking her to show you how she makes herself cum. It's a good way to learn what makes her feel good, too.

I want you to ride me right now.

Want your lady on top? Tell her to ride you hard and watch her jump on top.

I can't wait to bend you over the counter tonight.

A little verbal foreplay can go a long way, but this phrase works just as well in text as it does in person.

I can't wait to sink my dick into you.

Tell her how much you want to be inside her. It's a good way to heat things up between the two of you and get things going.

That makes you cream your panties, doesn't it?

Find something that really makes her squirm? Make sure she knows you know the power you hold over her.

Just look at how your little pussy opens up for my cock.

Telling her how she opens for you will make her feel like she belongs to you and you can use this to your advantage.

No one gets this pussy unless I say so.

Claiming her body and telling her that you have the right to say who gets to use it can be quite a heady feeling for both of you.

The more I finger you, the wetter you get. Tell me what you want.

Fingers are all find and good, but she really wants a hard dick in her vagina . . . but it's best to make her ask for it.

You're so wet! You want me to fuck you hard, don't you?

Commenting on her arousal can only result in more horniness in the long run, so go ahead and use it.

My cock feels so good in your tight little pussy.

This is a good phrase to use when you're barely moving, but fully sheathed inside her. It can really amp things up, but you get to choose when to move.

I'm going to leave my handprint on this pretty little ass.

This can be arousing and a warning that you're about to slap her pretty hard, hard enough to leave a mark.

When I'm around you, I just want to ravish your body.

You lose control around her and she should know that, especially if you want to have sex with her.

You look so hot and helpless when I pin you down like this.

Hold her hands above her head and tell her how sexy she looks to really get her squirming under you.

Let's hurry up and get home so I can get inside you before I explode.

Forget the date, just go home and fuck! She'll find it amazing that you want her that badly and skipping dessert won't be a problem.

Do you like my dick? Tell me how much you love it.

This is a great way to get her talking dirty to you and who doesn't want to hear hot stuff about his cock?

Tonight, I'm going to make you cum while you suck my fat cock.

Get her ready and thinking about what awaits her this evening. It's best to let her know early on so she can ruminate on it all day long and be nice and wet by nightfall.

Wear a skirt tonight so I can fuck you whenever and wherever I please.

Going out? Make sure she's in a skirt so you can feel her up while you are out and about. Just the thought of it will make her wet.

Pinch your nipples for me.

This will make her hot and it's pretty arousing to watch your lover turning herself on.

Open your legs and let's soak this bed.

She's going to have those legs spread wide in a moment, anticipating the wet antics that are about to follow.

Everywhere I go, I see furniture to bend you over.

This will let her know she's on your mind all the time and that having sex is also right up there with your other thoughts.

Filthy Phrases

This section is raunchy, but if you and your lady enjoy truly nasty dirty talk, then these phrases will turn you on like nobody's business. The big question though is, will it turn her on? These are no-holds barred kind of lines that will make her horny even if she thinks they're obscene and wrong. In fact, that's probably what will make her feel even more turned on.

I'm going to fuck you on the table/sofa/floor.

Let her know exactly what to expect from you and where it's going to happen. This can be used in the moment, or you can use it as foreplay.

I want to bang you so hard you forget you've ever been with anyone else.

This is a good way to start off some rough sex, if she's up for it. And she will certainly let you know if she is.

Your tight little pussy was made for my big dick.

Compliment her and give her pleasure as you dirty talk to her about your body parts.

I'm going to paint you from head to toe in my cream.

Don't just talk the big talk, make sure you do it just like you said. There's not much sexier than your woman drenched in hot cum.

I'm going to fuck a baby into you right now.

Whether or not you're actually trying for a baby, this phrase can really amp up the heat in the room and make her hornier than you ever thought.

I can't decide if I want to cum in your mouth or your pussy more.

This is a real turn on and she may have an opinion on where your cum should land, which makes for even more sexy talk.

You little slut, show me how wet you are for me.

This is a great way to turn both of you on even more. She'll get to open up to you and you can continue the sexy talk by describing how wet she is or what you're going to do with her.

This tight little pussy is my fuck toy tonight.

When you say this, she knows she's going to be used and abused by you all night long and that can be insanely hot.

I'm going to mark your breasts with love bites so everyone knows you're mine.

Marking your property can be very exciting for both of you and if she likes biting, you can do it even harder, preferably while pounding her at the same time.

I am destroying your tight cunt right now.

This is best said while you're going at it hard and fast. A little rough play goes well with some sex talk.

Cum all over my dick, baby, I want to see you squirt.

Female ejaculation isn't all that common, but if your girl can do it, let her know it's okay to go for it and that it will actually turn you on.

Shut up and take my dick in your tight pussy.

If you want silence instead of dirty talk, you can just tell her to shut up. When used in a sexual way, it can be very empowering.

You hungry, baby? Come here and I'll feed you my cock.

Domination can be very sexy and having her "eat" your penis is a fun way to make her obey you, plus it lets her know you want her to swallow.

Suck down every drop of my cum, I don't want a drop wasted.

Make sure she knows you want her to take everything you have to give and then some by telling her what to do with your cum.

I'm going to spurt so deep inside you that you won't stop cumming for a week.

Telling her what you're going to do to her sexually, especially when it indicates being rather out of control, can be very exciting for both of you.

Fuck me like a porn star.

Not only will you make her feel sexy, you'll make her feel like an actual porn star with this phrase.

I need to go down on you, I've been craving your pussy all day.

She'll be eager to get into bed when you use this line on her and it shows that she's important to you . . . since you're craving her.

Who owns this fucking pussy? Tell me!

Dominance can be a real turn on, so don't be afraid to use it and if she responds well, take it even further.

Those sweet lips deserve to get fucked.

What do you want to do to her? Tell her by telling her how she deserves it and even why she does.

I want you gagging on my cock.

Violent talk is not for everyone, but this mildly sexual version can be just harsh enough to kick your evening into extra hot mode.

Ride me like you mean it, baby.

You can tell her how to ride you, suggest she go faster, harder, etc. but just telling your girl to ride you like she means it will result in all those things.

Act like the little slut you are.

Want to get down and dirty? Call her a slut or whore. This is not for everyone, so be sure she is into it before you start talking like this.

This pussy is mine, all mine. I own it.

Claim her as yours and you'll both be turned on. This is a common theme in romance books and something that women tend to enjoy greatly.

I can't wait any longer, I'm going to fuck you right here and I don't care who sees.

Urgency shows her that you can't handle waiting any longer because she is just so sexy.

I'm going to cum all over your tits/pussy/ass.

The act of ejaculating on your partner is exhilarating, but it's even more so when you announce your intentions to mark her.

I'm going to cum so hard. I'm going to knock you up.

Even if you're practicing safe sex, dirty talking about getting her pregnant can really amp things up for you.

I'm going to fuck you until you can't even walk.

This is another slightly violent phrase, but it will get her wet faster than anything else you can say, imagining how hard you're going to work her over.

Keep talking dirty, girl and I'm going to wash your mouth out with my cum.

You can encourage her to keep mouthing off, while turning it into a sexy way to dirty talk and a fun finish.

The thought of your hot mouth on my hard cock makes me so horny.

You're not actually telling her to do it, but by providing a mental image of what you want, you can give her a little nudge in the right direction.

Your ass looks so great while I'm fucking this little pussy from behind.

This can be accompanied by a slap or two on said ass if you are so inclined and you know she likes it.

Suck my hard dick while I eat you out.

Ready for some 69? Turn it into a dirty command and she'll be on board.

I wish I could fuck your pussy and your mouth at the same time.

This will give her a hint of how hard it is to choose a hole. Of course, if she's up for a threesome, you can actually manage this.

Your cunt is gripping my dick so hard right now.

You can feel it and so can she, but hearing it will make her cum even harder, which will result in more gripping.

Where do you want me to cum, pussy or ass?

Give her the choice . . . since you'll enjoy it either way.

I can't wait until we get home, let's find a closet so I can fuck you right now.

When you're out on a date or anywhere that is public, this will have her scouring the location for a spot to get you off.

This pussy is so tight, I might break it.

She'll really be turned on as you take things up a notch and start pounding her right after you say this.

DIRTY TALK FOR WOMEN

If you're looking to make your guy horny and know that dirty talk turns him on, then this is the section for you. Men love to hear that you like what they do, so they're going to particularly enjoy phrases that compliment their size, prowess, and let them know that they're making you hot. But there's no reason you can't use this dirty talk to turn yourself on, too!

Mild Dirty Talk

To start out, you might want to keep things fairly mild. These phrases work for anyone, whether they enjoy serious dirty talk or just want to hear a little bit about how much you want them. If you're feeling a bit shy about talking sexily, then you can start out with these simpler phrases and lines.

Damn, your ass looks good in those jeans.

Men enjoy compliments on what they're wearing and he'll be happy that his butt turns you on.

You enjoying the view? Good, because it's all yours.

This phrase can be accompanied by a little spin or by running your hands down your body to emphasis your curves.

Let me take care of you tonight.

Let your nurturing side come out and give him everything he's looking for. It's a fun method of taking control without being too dominant.

I want you inside me.

Something every man wants to hear is how much you need him inside you. This phrase is practically guaranteed to get him even more excited.

You make me think such dirty things.

He has that kind of effect on you, so let him know. Chances are, he'll want you to elaborate.

Guess what I'm wearing?

Everyone knows the old favorite . . . asking a lady what she's wearing. In this case, you're taking charge and making him guess.

I have whipped cream and chocolate sauce. Come lick it off me.

Adding food to the sex routine can be a lot of fun and it makes for an extra luscious booty call.

I love how big and strong you are.

Men enjoy physical compliments just as much as women and telling him how strong he is will help him feel even sexier in bed.

When you kiss my neck/breasts/earlobe, I get all tingly.

Give him a picture of what you feel when he's loving on you and get more explicit if it sounds like he's enjoying what you're saying.

This morning, I was wet just thinking about you.

He'll love knowing that your body reacts to him even when he's not actually there.

I want you to touch me here.

Show him exactly what you want and you'll both have an amazing time. This is a good place to grab his hand and put it where you want him touching you.

Do you like it when I touch myself like this?

Men love to see a woman masturbate, so go ahead and pleasure yourself, giving him little teasers as you go. This can be done in person or you can send him a photo or video.

You're so big!

Complimenting him on his size will always go over well, too.

You get so hard when I _____.

Whatever you're doing, keep it up . . . and tell him straight out that you notice his reaction.

I got new lingerie, wanna see?

He'll definitely want to see and the fact that you got something new to show off to him will be icing on the cake.

Your hard dick is really turning me on.

Men are always up for compliments on their dicks and when you let him know how much it turns you on, he'll be raring to go.

I'm not wearing any panties.

This is best used when you're out and about and he can't actually do anything about the fact that you're naked under your dress. It will keep him thinking about you until he can check for himself.

How can someone so strong be so gentle?

If you're not feeling the rough stuff tonight, just break out this line and watch him treat you like a china doll.

There's nowhere I'd rather be than on top of you.

When you want to ride your guy, this is a nice clear way of letting him know while still being seductive.

You better get in here before I start without you.

When he needs a little boost to get him moving, whether he's in the shower, or still at work, you can get him going with a simple suggestion like this. Just thinking about you touching yourself will have him horny and ready to go.

Spank me harder!

Step things up a bit with more spanking, if you enjoy it. If you love it, he'll probably love it, too.

Get over here and feel just how wet you make me.

Try this one in a crowded place to get the excitement up a little. He can secretively feel you up and then you can escape to a more private area to bang.

My pussy misses your dick.

Short, sweet, and to the point. He'll definitely take measures to remedy this particular problem. A good phrase for long distance courting.

Dirty Talk

Ready to take it up to the next level? Men tend to enjoy raunchy talk and these lines will get him hard fast! As you become more confident in your ability to turn him on, you can use these hot lines to really make him ready for you. They will probably turn you on, too.

Your dick feels so good inside me.

Take this one a step further and describe how it feels to have him inside you, using sensory words like slick, thick, or stimulating.

You've turned me into such a little slut.

He'll feel awesome that his sex has made you crave it more. This is also good motivation for him to keep sexing you up properly.

Oh, you're stretching me out so much!

This is another way of telling him that he's big. You might want to follow up by describing just how amazing it feels.

Lean back and let me take care of that hard on for you.

It looks a little painful to be that hard so why not help a guy out? Give him permission to relax while you go down on him.

See how wet I am? Don't you want to get up in here?

Show him how wet you are and invite him to slide right on in to really turn him on.

I get soaked when you're so rough with me.

He'll be even rougher after you tell him this, so only say it if you're good with that.

I soaked my panties and it's all your fault.

This phrase is best used when you're out and about or in a restaurant, to make him hard in public.

Grab my tits, baby.

If you like breast play and he's not giving you enough of it, you need to be nice and direct.

I want to suck your cock while you lick my pussy.

Get him in the mood for 69ing with this sexy phrase and you'll be enjoying hot, dirty oral sex in no time.

Suck me harder, it feels so good.

Whether his mouth is on your clit or your breast, you can encourage him to step up the suckling very easily.

You know just how to eat my pussy.

If he's good at oral, then make sure you let him know that he's doing a good job. After all, that's a rare thing in this world and you want to keep him down there.

I want your mouth on my tits.

Give him specific directions to turn you on and he'll be more than happy to give you what you want.

I need your mouth on my clit right now.

If you've been thinking of this all day and need a little extra something to get turned on, this is a great way to let him know.

I've been thinking of getting on my knees for you since this morning.

Blow jobs are awfully hot for a guy and the fact that you've been thinking about it all day will get him hard instantly.

You get harder and I get wetter.

Your bodies are linked through the sex act, so make a comment on how wet it makes you to see him getting harder.

I can't wait to feel your big cock inside my wet pussy.

A little dirty talk can go a long way when it comes to men and this one is a phrase he'll be revisiting frequently whenever he thinks of sex with you.

Not sure what makes me hornier, your ____ or your _____.

He'll feel super sexy when you can't decide which part of his body is the hottest. Pick any two parts . . . and they don't necessarily have to be genitals.

I want that big hard dick in my mouth right now.

He'll be more than happy to make your dream come true when you talk to him like this.

I'm going to suck on these big balls until you're begging to be inside me.

Don't just go for the obvious sex organs when you're getting hot and bothered . . . experiment and try out a few different techniques.

I love having you so deep inside me.

Make him feel amazing by complimenting how deep he can go, no matter his size. It will turn him on more and make him want to thrust even deeper.

I'm your sex slave for the night. Tell me what you want.

You'll fulfill his fantasies and make him extra horny when you offer yourself up to him for the night.

I just want to worship your cock. It's so perfect.

This is the perfect phrase to offer up before you start giving him a blow job. Tell him you want to worship it, then do it.

I'm going to lick you until you come and then I'm going to lap up all your jizz.

If he doesn't get harder just hearing how you're going to make him cum and then eat up his juice, you might need a new partner.

Tie me up and fuck me senseless.

He's going to love tying you up, but this command is also giving him control over you, making it really hot.

Cum in my mouth so I can taste that heavenly liquid.

What guy doesn't love to ejaculate in a woman's mouth? Tell him upfront that you want it and watch out for the explosion.

I love it when you take control like this.

If you enjoy being dominated, you can encourage even a not-so-dominant guy to take charge by telling him how much you like it.

Sucking your dick is my favorite part of the day.

Dreaming all day of wrapping your lips around him? Then go ahead and tell him, either before you meet up or as you're about to go down on him.

I want you to kiss me after you go down on me, I love tasting myself on you.

Not only does this encourage him to go down on you, it also makes him anticipate giving you your own juices, which is pretty darn hot.

Fill me up with your big cock.

You want him inside you and this is a great way to tell him to do it right now.

I'm going to cum so hard if you keep this up.

Want him to keep going? Then tell him just how very hard you'll explode all over him and he'll keep doing what he's doing.

Mmm, your dick tastes so good.

He'll immediately get harder when you moan this phrase at him. Anything that praises his penis will get a rise.

I've never seen you this hard, baby, let's put it to good use.

Once you've made him extra horny with your dirty talk, let him know that you intend to make use of his erection.

Give me that load, all over my face/tits!

Tell him to cum on you and he'll likely oblige! This kind of talk can really turn a guy on and it might be just what he needs to put him over the edge.

Do you love my juicy pussy?

This gives him an opportunity to carry the dirty talk torch and tell you just how much he loves your pussy.

Come on, baby, pound me into oblivion.

If you want it harder, this is a fun, sexy way to get him to really give it to you.

You're the only man who could make me feel this good.

He'll get even harder, knowing he's the only one for you. It's a great phrase to use in the middle of sex, especially if he's in control.

I want to taste myself on your fingers.

Give him a really good reason to finger you with this erotic talk. He'll be diving in as fast as he can.

You're a fucking sex god.

Any man would be thrilled to hear this and it will boost his ego so much, he'll want to please you all night long.

I can already tell I'm going to cum more than once tonight.

If you tend to have multiple orgasms, let him know right out that you intend to thoroughly enjoy yourself with him. Plus, he'll strive to make you cum more than once.

I've been waiting for your dick my whole life.

Is he an amazing lover? Tell him how incredible his cock is and what you want to do with it.

Let me ride you so you can suck my tits while I fuck you.

Take charge with specific directions and make both of you feel amazing.

Do you like watching me finger myself?

Watching a woman masturbate is pretty pleasurable for the guy, too, so go ahead and pleasure yourself and make him watch, talking dirty the whole time.

I bet I can make you cum in less than five minutes, using only my mouth.

Challenge accepted! He'll certainly want to take this bet, but chances are, he'll lose, which means you get to pick your prize.

My ass had better be bright red in the morning.

Encourage him to smack you but good with this kind of dirty talk. Tell him how much it turns you on, too.

I had sexy panties on, but they got too wet, so I had to take them off.

This is a terrific teaser that will get him all hot and bothered. It's a good thing to tell him while you're out on a date, or at a formal ceremony.

I want you to squirt in me so bad.

This gives him the mental image of cumming inside you without any protection, which is definitely a turn on.

Filthy Phrases

If you feel like going even further into the dirty talk, these phrases will help you move things along pretty quickly. They are also very useful if you want something specific or if you're in need of some rough and hard sex. You can let him know pretty quickly that you're up for whatever he wants to try.

I want you to fuck my tits and cum on my face.

With such a vivid word picture, who could resist? Probably not your guy.

I could tell you how horny I am, but I'd rather you stick your fingers in my pussy and feel for yourself.

This is a longer sentence to use, but it will get the desired result and fast. He'll be inside you in a moment.

No foreplay tonight, just get your dick inside me. Now.

Foreplay is nice and all, but if you're already horny, you can get him in the mood in a split second by telling him that you're ready to go right now.

I want to milk you for every drop of cum you have to give me.

You can use this for oral sex or vaginal. Either one will get him gushing into you faster than ever before.

I'm going to sit on your face until I can't cum anymore.

Just let him know what is in store for him and then fulfill your mission. Don't forget to repay the favor once he's done.

You aren't doing anything else/anymore work tonight until you cum in my mouth.

He'll gladly give up whatever he's been doing to take you up on your generous offer and it could even turn into a full-blown roll in the hay.

Cum inside me and then I'm going to lick your dick clean.

This will get him harder and hornier than ever, thinking of you cleaning your mutual juices off of his penis.

Suck my baby cock like you're going to make me cum in your mouth.

Your clit may not be capable of squirting all over him, but you can surely try to make it happen.

I want to feel your cum dripping out of me.

He'll love to brand you with his semen and the thought of it filling you to overflowing will be more than enough to get him hard.

Tonight, I'm just your dirty little slut. Use me as you will.

Turn the control over to him and make him feel special as you worship his body.

I want you to fuck me so hard I can't walk tomorrow.

This will definitely get him aroused and you'll probably have some of the best sex ever.

I want it rough tonight. Give it to me hard.

If you're up for something a bit rougher than normal, make sure you let him in on the secret. Chances are, he'll be more than thrilled to get a bit rowdier.

I'm going to lick your cock until it's as soaked as my pussy.

You can use this as a jumping off point for a lot more sexy talk. What are you going to do with that cock once it's all wet?

No one has ever fucked me like this before.

Make him really feel like a sex god by telling him how incredible he is and how you've never felt this way before.

I'm a cock/cum hungry slut, are you going to feed me?

He'll be in a rush to get his dick in you when you mention how crazy you are for it. You can change this phrase up with any word for penis and he'll go crazy.

Oh yeah, I'm going to squirt all over your cock/face!

Whether or not you can squirt, just the thought of it will be enough to make him harder than ever.

Where do you want to cum, baby?

Giving him a choice will immediately get his mind racing as he imagines the possibilities.

Make me your little cum slut, daddy.

You can drop the daddy part if you wish, but telling him to basically make you his slave can only turn him on more.

Make me scream with your big cock!

Telling a guy his penis is big is always a good way to go. Telling him how to use it is even better.

I want to be your love slave. Do me now.

This will give him all kinds of ideas and he'll be dirty talking sooner, rather than later. After all, he'd be crazy to turn down a sex slave.

You think you can get your cock in me without anyone seeing?

Even if you don't actually do it, this comment in a public place will get his mind racing with all the possibilities.

Take me from behind and fuck me silly.

Love being fucked from behind? He'll love it too, especially when you put it this way.

You better clean up all those juices you just shot into me, with your mouth.

Take control and make him go down on you after he's come. Just because he had his fun doesn't mean yours is over.

I can't wait to lick your cock clean.

First, make him come, then clean him up. He'll love hearing all about it with this dirty talk.

I want you in every one of my holes.

This will let him know you're up for just about anything and lets him know that all your orifices are open to him.

I want to grind my pussy into your face.

Thinking of riding his face? This is a sexy way to tell him what you have in mind. He'll probably be all for it!

Put that big fat baby maker in me now!

Certain words can really set the mood and while you can switch out baby maker with any penis word, this one is likely to make him extra hard.

Fuck me from behind like a dog.

Want to do it doggy style? Let him know with some nasty talk.

I can't wait to taste your cum on my lips.

He'll love hearing these words on your lips and will want to give you exactly what you want.

Fuck me harder!

Most men will happily oblige and if you're close to the edge, this is a good way to let him know what will make you feel even better.

I want your cum all over me/my breasts.

Give him permission to ejaculate all over you or specific body parts and just the thought of it will make him hornier.

Your prick is the perfect fit inside me.

He's going to love hearing that he fits you perfectly and makes you feel ever so amazing, so go ahead and tell him.

My pussy is going to suck every last drop of cum out of you.

If you're feeling feisty, jump on your man and tell him you're going to milk him for all he's got. It's bound to make him hot.

You want this pussy? Come and get it, big boy.

This one is best used as you crawl away from him, or lead him to your desired location for having sex.

Pound my cunt harder!

These are words that will get him pumping harder than ever.

I want you in my ass right now.

Anal sex isn't for everyone, but if you enjoy it, let your man know that you want him in your ass and he'll be raring to go.

Yes, baby, give me all your hot, delicious cum!

For blow jobs, if you want him to cum in your mouth, you should let him know before he blows his load, but this phrase works equally well before or during.

Use me like I'm your precious fuck toy.

This sentence gives him permission to do what he wishes, which can be a heady experience for both of you and a fun way to experiment with limits.

I just came thinking about you, but if you get here fast, we can go for round two.

He'll be psyched that you masturbated to him, but the idea of getting to you quickly, before the heat cools down will have him running out the door.

Fuck my face!

There are blow jobs and there are face fuckings. If the latter is what you want, then tell him to get on with it.

I'm your little whore.

Feeling dirty? He'll probably love it when you not only offer yourself up as his, but also as a bad girl. You can use this to lead into being punished, if you so desire.

Destroy my pussy! Take it all.

If you want it rough, then you need to tell your lover and this particular nasty phase will get you exactly what you want.

I can feel you filling me up with your hot cum.

Dirty talk in the middle of an orgasm is a great way to take the high to even higher peaks. Go ahead and try it and you'll see.

All I could think about all day is how I want to gag on your cock.

He'll be ready for a blow job in seconds if you start talking to him like this. Then be prepared for some deep throating.

I want you to cum inside me this time.

Giving him permission to ejaculate inside you is a good way to make sure he gets hard and stays that way.

I'm your little cum bucket, fill me up.

The ultimate in dirty talk will make him want to ejaculate all over you in no time flat.

I'm going to suck you dry before you leave for work.

He won't be able to resist this particular sexy talk and you'll have a dick in your mouth before you know it.

You can fuck any hole you want tonight.

Give him an open invitation with this phrase and you'll drive him crazy. He won't know where to start!

POST-COITAL DIRTY TALK

If you're in a long term relationship, don't miss out on the opportunity to use some dirty talk the day after you've had mind-blowing sex. It may even end up being foreplay for more awesome sex later on.

Last night was so hot, I can't wait for a repeat.

Reliving the previous night's sex is a surefire way to get riled up for the next round, so make sure your partner is thinking about it, too.

I can't even concentrate at work, last night keeps running through my mind.

Who doesn't want to be an incredible distraction? Let your lover know exactly what effect they had on you.

That was the most unbelievable sex I've ever had.

Remind them that you were blown away by their sexual abilities the night before and you'll have a repeat in no time.

Can't stop thinking about how hot you were last night.

Want to get them hot again? Keep talking about how amazing they were the night before.

You were so amazing yesterday, I still feel weak-kneed.

Admiring the sexual prowess of your lover is always a good way to go the next day.

I can hardly walk today. You were so incredible.

This is a surefire way to make someone feel like they did a good job, but be sure to reassure them that they were amazing after you mention how damaged you are from the sex!

Are you as exhausted as I am from that incredible orgasm last night?

Share your exhaustion with your partner. If things were as amazing as you thought, they're still thinking about it, too.

I can still feel your juices/cum on me.

Knowing you left your scent on your lover can be intoxicating, so this phrase works well in letting them know you're still thinking of them.

I'm so sore from last night, but in the best way possible.

This works best for women, but a guy can be sore from the sexual acrobatics, as well. Either way, it's a great reminder of why you want to get together again.

COMING UP WITH YOUR OWN PHRASES

While there are more than enough dirty talk ideas in this book to get you started, you might still find that nothing really clicks that well with you. That's fine, since you should be coming up with your own dirty phrases anyway. How do you do that? It's surprisingly easy.

There are a few ways to approach this:

Admire the Body

First, look at what you love about your partner. What body parts stand out to you? You probably have a few favorites and not just their genitals.

Now, consider what you want to do to that body part. Are you longing to kiss it, lick it, suck it, or fondle it? Go ahead and tell your lover that. Describe in detail what you plan to do to them. You're already talking dirty and it's all you.

Try flipping this around and telling your lover exactly what you want them to do or what you love about them doing things to your own body parts. For example, you might say, "It's so sexy when you lick my chest like that."

Bring On the Fantasies

Another option is to fantasize about how you'd like to screw your lover. What moves do you want to try? Where do you fantasize about fucking them (even if you would never really do it, talking about it is sexy)? Do you fantasize about adding another person to the mix?

Talk your fantasies out, but keep it short and to the point. For example, instead of expounding on how much you'd love a threesome, say something like, "You're so fucking sexy, I wish there were two of you." Or "If we had another guy here, he could go down on me while I suck your dick." Just the images that these words conjure up is often enough to really heat things up.

Use All Senses

Usually, we say things like, "that feels so good" or "you taste so good." These are phrases that use senses, but most people focus on just touch and sight. Try to incorporate every sense into your dirty talk. Tell them how their scent turns you on and how sweet they taste. Tell them that you love the little panting noises and moans that they make when you touch them in a certain way.

Try blending multiple senses into one sentence to really create a vivid mind picture that will really get their juices flowing.

Focus On Their Turn On

What does your partner like most in the opposite sex? A little observation can tell you a lot about what they love, but you can also just ask. A few questions to get things flowing:

What's your favorite body part on a man/woman?

What sexual position have you always wanted to try?

What is your hottest fantasy?

What porn move do you wish you could experience?

This will give you more ideas for talking dirty next time you're in bed together.

Give Commands

Getting all masterful and dominant isn't for everyone, but it can sure make for some fun sexy times. It also ensures you get exactly what you need to reach orgasm.

Tell your partner what to do, but in a forceful manner. It can help if you imagine being a drill sergeant in charge of bringing you both to orgasm. This works very well for both sexes and can really be a turn on for both sides. Saying something like, "Bite my neck right now!" can turn the heat up to 10 in a second.

There's no shortage of ways to come up with your very own sexy phrases, so get creative and let the sexual high take you to new places.

FINAL THOUGHTS

Now you have plenty of weapons in your arsenal, so it's time to get out there and start using them.